The Complete Metabolism Diet

The following Book is reproduced below with the goal of providing information that is as accurate and reliable as possible. Regardless, purchasing this Book can be seen as consent to the fact that both the publisher and the author of this book are in no way experts on the topics discussed within and that any recommendations or suggestions that are made herein are for entertainment purposes only. Professionals should be consulted as needed prior to undertaking any of the action endorsed herein.

This declaration is deemed fair and valid by both the American Bar Association and the Committee of Publishers Association and is legally binding throughout the United States.

Furthermore, the transmission, duplication or reproduction of any of the following work including specific information will be considered an illegal act irrespective of if it is done electronically or in print. This extends to creating a secondary or tertiary copy of the work or a recorded copy and is only allowed with an expressed written consent from the Publisher. All additional right reserved.

The information in the following pages is broadly considered to be a truthful and accurate account of facts, and as such any inattention, use or misuse of the information in question by the reader will render any resulting actions solely under their purview. There are no scenarios in which the publisher or the original author of this work can be in any fashion deemed liable for any hardship or damages that may befall them after undertaking information described herein.

Additionally, the information in the following pages is intended only for informational purposes and should thus be thought of as universal. As befitting its nature, it is presented without assurance regarding its prolonged validity or interim quality. Trademarks that are mentioned are done without written consent and can in no way be considered an endorsement from the trademark holder.

Table of Contents

Introduction

Congratulations on purchasing *The Complete Metabolism Diet* and thank you for doing so. The world of diet is growing increasingly, and downloading this book is the first step you can take towards actually doing something about transitioning to a healthful diet. The first step is also not always the easiest, which is why it is important to take the information you will find in the following chapters seriously for they are not concepts that can be put into action immediately. If you keep these concepts in file, when the time comes to actually use them, you will be glad that you have them at hand.

To that end, the following chapters will discuss the primary preparedness principles that you need to consider if you ever decide to realistically be ready for losing weight and gaining health with a Complete Metabolism Diet. This means that you will need to consider the quality of your food including the potential issues raised by their quality, how they can best be utilized in a meal, and various tools you might need to keep your mind focused on the task at hand.

With quality out of the way, you will then learn everything you need to know about preparing a wide variety of recipes including common fruit and vegetable recipes along with less common dishes as well.

I am happy to welcome you to the world of dieting and to help you lose weight, change your life, and become a healthier person.

BONUS:

As a way of saying thank you for purchasing my book, please use your link below to claim your 3 FREE Cookbooks on Health, Fitness & Dieting Instantly

https://bit.ly/2MkqTit

You can also share your link with your friends and families whom you think that can benefit from the cookbooks or you can forward them the link as a gift!

Chapter 1: Week 1

Day 1

Ricotta cake with pears

Ingredients:

- 100 gr of ricotta
- 50 gr of sugar
- 2 vanilla seeds
- 3 eggs
- 1 package of baking powder

Preparation

1. To prepare the soft ricotta cake and pears, start by peeling the pears. Then, remove the central core and cut them into small cubes.
2. Place them in a bowl with very little lemon juice to prevent them from browning. Mix the sugar with the ricotta.
3. Then, add the seeds of the vanilla bean. Then, add 3 eggs one by one and continue to whisk the mixture.
4. Add the grated lemon peel. Sift the flour with the baking powder and add it to the mixture while stirring with a wooden spoon until you get a smooth dough. Stir in the diced pears and mix them with the dough.
5. Grease and flour a 24 cm diameter cake pan. Pour the cake dough and level it with a spatula. Bake the cake at 180 ° C (static oven) for 50 to 70 minutes. If the cake gets too dark on the surface, cover it with aluminum foil.
6. Take out the soft ricotta and pear pie from the oven, let it cool, shake it, and sprinkle with icing sugar before serving!

Chicken and avocado

Ingredients

- 100 gr of chicken
- 1 avocado
- ½ lemon
- 60 gr of oil

Preparation

1. For the recipe of chicken and avocado salad with ginger sauce, fry the chicken meat and set it aside in a bowl.
2. Peel the ginger and grate it. Then, squeeze the ginger pulp in your hands and pour the juice into a small bowl; add the juice of 1/2 lemon, 60 g of oil, a pinch of salt and parsley and blend in a dipping mixer to obtain a sauce.
3. Clean the avocado and cut into chunks. Season the chicken with the ginger sauce and top with avocado chunks. To make it taste better, you can also add the peeled lemon segments to add zesty flavor.

Pasta with broccoli

Ingredients

- 150 gr of pasta
- 50 gr broccoli
- salt
- parmesan cheese, if you like it

Preparation

1. To prepare pasta with broccoli, you must first wash and cut the vegetables. Then, sauté them in a pan with garlic and oil.
2. Meanwhile, cook the pasta in boiling salted water. Once the

pasta has reached its al dente state, drain it. Season it with the broccoli.

3. Stir in everything and add a bit of cheese. This cheese will represent the final touch of your dish and will give more creaminess to your pasta with broccoli. Mix it again. For the final steps, serve the dish and if you like it, add a little bit more cheese.

Day 2

Cocoa and mint

Ingredients

- 100 gr of coconut butter
- 50 gr of coconut
- 1 tablespoon of coconut oil
- cocoa powder

Preparation

1. Cocoa and mint are an excellent combination, and they are perfect for the complete metabolism diet. Let's see this recipe.
2. Combine 100 grams of melted coconut butter, 50 grams of grated coconut, 1 tablespoon of coconut oil and half a teaspoon of peppermint extract. Mix well and pour into cream puffs or muffin molds, filling them halfway. Place in the fridge to harden (about 15 minutes).
3. Mix 2 tablespoons of melted coconut oil and 2 tablespoons of cocoa powder. Retrieve the peppermint mixture from the refrigerator and pour the cocoa mixture into each mold over the peppermint. Refrigerate until the bombs harden.
4. Before serving, remove the bombs from the refrigerator and let them rest for about 5 minutes.

Cesar salad

Ingredients

- fresh salad
- bread
- 10gr of butter
- 1 egg
- ½ lemon
- parmesan cheese

Preparation

1. To prepare the Caesar salad, wash, dry, and finely cut the Romaine salad and place it in a large bowl.
2. Cut the bread into cubes. Melt the butter in a frying pan and pour in the cubes of bread until they are brown and crunchy.
3. Prepare the sauce with the aid of a food processor: pour the egg, lemon juice, white vinegar, peeled garlic, and Worcestershire sauce into the glass of the food processor; begin to blend and add the oil little by little, then flush until you get a consistency similar to mayonnaise.
4. Add the cubes of Parmesan cheese and crispy bread to the salad. Then, season with the freshly prepared sauce. Serve your well-seasoned and mixed Caesar salad.

Tasty Rolls

Ingredients

- 100 gr of chicken
- 1 mozzarella
- pepper
- salt

Preparation

1. To prepare your rolls, start by slightly flattening the chicken slices with the meat tenderizer. Take a slice of chicken and place a slice of mozzarella cheese on it.
2. Roll the slice on itself to get some rolls and fix them with a toothpick. Spice up each roll with a tuft of rosemary. Heat the oil in a pan and place the rolls in it, adding salt and pepper, and cook for about 15 minutes in total. Halfway through cooking, add the juice of half a lemon and let it evaporate. Serve the rolls when they are still hot.

Day 3

Morning Donuts

Ingredients

- 200 gr of flour
- 1 package of baking powder
- 50 gr of butter
- 1 egg
- 50 gr of sugar
- Salt

Preparation

1. To make the morning donuts, start by mixing the flour and baking powder, sieving everything in a large bowl.
2. Grate the rind of an orange that will serve to flavor the dough. Separately, in another bowl put the butter softened and reduced into small pieces, add the sugar and whip the mixture with electric whips to get a cream.
3. At this point add the whole egg and the yolk at room temperature, and a pinch of salt. Continue by assembling the mixture with the whips and, with the whips in action, pour the milk at room temperature. Add the powders to the mixture of eggs and butter a little at a time, helping with a spoon.
4. Then mix with electric whips until a smooth and lumpy mixture is obtained. Take a donuts mold, butter the bottom and edges of the mold with a kitchen brush. To better butter the entire surface, a fundamental precaution if you use a decorated mold like that that we used. Finally, sprinkle the whole surface of the mold with flour.
5. Pour the mixture into the pan and level the surface with a spatula or the back of a spoon. Cook the morning donuts in a preheated oven at 170 degrees for 40 minutes. When cooked,

take the donuts out and let it cool before taking it out.

6. In a bowl mix the powdered sugar with the powdered cinnamon, then sprinkle the mixture of aromas on the cake.

Lemon spaghetti

Ingredients

- 150 gr of spaghetti
- 1 lemon
- 10 gr of butter

Preparation

1. To prepare spaghetti with lemon, place a pot with plenty of slightly salted water on the stove; as soon as it boils, cook the spaghetti according to the package directions.
2. In a pan melt the butter, add the lemon and stir for two minutes, then add the juice.
3. In a separate pan, toast the pine nuts taking care that they do not burn, then wash and dry the basil.
4. Drain the pasta keeping a glass of cooking water, add it to the lemon juice and mix well until it is all blended.
5. Add the Ricotta and a ladle of cooking water and mix well until it has formed a velvety cream that wraps the spaghetti.

Fried anchovies

Ingredients

- 50 gr of anchovies
- 100 gr of corn flour
- 1 mozzarella
- olive oil as much as you want
- salt

Preparation

1. The preparation of fried anchovies is easy, fast and suitable for every situation.
2. We start by sifting the cornflour with the white flour and the powdered (very finely grated) lemon peel.
3. Cut the green part of the courgettes into julienne strips; with the potato peeler cut the remaining part and finally cut thin sticks of mozzarella cheese. Then, roll the anchovies and open them to book, dry them and fill them with a stick of mozzarella cheese and a few slices of zucchini.
4. Finish the preparation of fried anchovies by closing and wrapping them in a courgette ribbon, pass them in lemon flour and fry in plenty of extra virgin olive oil. When cooked, it is advisable to drain them and place them on a layer of absorbent paper. Salt the fried anchovies and serve them hot.

Day 4

Oatmeal

Ingredients

- 100 gr of oatmeal
- 1 egg
- 50 gr of flour
- chocolate

Preparation

1. Put the oatmeal into a mixer. In a large saucepan melt the butter gently, turn off the heat and add the oatmeal and mix well. Cut the oat flakes in a mixer. In a large pot gently melt the butter, turn off the heat, add the oatmeal and mix well.
2. In a bowl mounted with electric whips, mix the egg with the granulated and whole sugar until you have a well-assembled mixture. It will take about 2 minutes. Add the flour sifted with baking powder and continue to assemble. Add the oatmeal and mix well with a wooden spoon. At the end add the chocolate, leaving some aside for the final decoration, and mix until the mixture is homogeneous.
3. With the help of a teaspoon spread the mixture on a baking sheet covered with parchment paper. Make lots of small piles of compost trying to give a round shape, you can help with the back of a slightly wet teaspoon or if you want to be more precise use a cookie cutter of 5 cm in diameter and with a teaspoon press the mixture until you have so many pods, put on the chocolate drops kept aside. Spread them well because they tend to spread out during cooking.

Caprese

Ingredients

- salad
- tuna
- tomatoes
- mozzarella
- olive oil 10 gr

Preparation

1. To prepare the Caprese salad with tuna, wash the tomatoes well, dry them and cut them into wedges; then cut the mozzarella cheese into slices that are not too thin.
2. Drain the tuna, then wash and dry the salads well and place them on a serving dish in the center where you put the tuna and all around the slices of tomato and mozzarella cheese.
3. In a separate bowl, prepare a mixture of capers, basil, and anchovies: add salt and white pepper, then pour the balsamic vinegar and mix well until it mixes.
4. Serve your tuna Caprese salad with the freshly prepared sauce and a drizzle of extra virgin olive oil.

Fresh salad

Ingredients

- valerian salad
- 1 apple
- 1 certosa cheese
- salt
- pepper
- balsamic vinegar
- oil

Preparation

1. Put the valerian on the bottom of the saucers, cover it with thin slices of apple and small portions of Certosa Light. Sauté the speck into small pieces and spread it warm on the salad and season with an emulsion of oil, salt, pepper and balsamic vinegar.

Day 5

Pancakes

Ingredients

- baking soda
- 100 gr of flour
- 1 package of baking powder
- 2 tablespoons of cream
- 2 tablespoons of milk
- 2 tablespoons of chocolate cream
- fresh fruit

Preparation

1. In a bowl, sift the flour with baking soda and salt and add the sugar, baking powder and egg. Mix with the whisk
2. Pour the milk and continue to mix until the batter is obtained. Then add a generous teaspoon of custard cream and mix well. Pour the milk and continue to mix until the batter is obtained.
3. For the sauce: add 2 tablespoons of cream and 2 tablespoons of milk and heat in a saucepan (or in the microwave). Add more milk according to the density that you like and pour into a small dairy. For the sauce: add 2 tablespoons of chocolate cream and 2 tablespoons of milk and heat in a saucepan (or in the microwave). Add more milk depending on the density that you like and pour it into a small dairy.
4. Stack the pancakes to taste and serve with the hazelnut sauce garnishing with fresh fruit.

Spaghetti with bottarga

Ingredients

- 150 gr of spaghetti
- 20 gr of bottarga
- salt
- 10 gr of butter

Preparation

1. To prepare spaghetti with bottarga, cook the spaghetti in plenty of not too salty water.
2. Meanwhile, heat the marsala in a pan just by evaporating the alcohol; remove from heat and add the butter. Drain the spaghetti well and stir in the Marsala and the butter. Add the bottarga, a sprinkling of breadcrumbs and mix well.
3. Serve your spaghetti with hot bottarga.

Pasta and mozzarella

Ingredients

- 150 gr of pasta
- 1 mozzarella
- 1 tomato
- olive oil
- capers

Preparation

1. To prepare your pasta with mozzarella follow us in these few simple steps: take a pot with high sides and cook the pasta.
2. In the meantime, take the mozzarella cheese and cut it into slices in a bowl.
3. Do the same with the tomato, cutting it into wedges.

4. Now add a little oil and for those who want a handful of capers and anchovy paste.
5. Once cooked the pasta, drain it and pour it into the tureen with the rest of the ingredients.
6. Mix everything and decorate with basil leaves.

Day 6
Brioche without dough

Ingredients

- 20 gr of butter
- 200 gr of flour
- 1 package of baking powder
- 100 gr of milk

Preparation

1. This brioche without dough is ready in 5 minutes: just mix the ingredients with a fork, let it rest for 24 hours and then cook it. A minimum effort for a great result! Excellent alone or with jam, it is perfect for breakfast or as a snack.
2. Melt the butter and let it cool. Pour the flour into a bowl, add the baking powder, sugar, and salt. Stir, then incorporate the eggs, the melted butter and finally the milk. Stir quickly with a fork, cover with the food foil and leave to rise for 3 hours at room temperature, in a warm place and away from drafts.
3. After this time, transfer the dough in the refrigerator and let it rest for 24 hours.
4. Before baking the brioche, leave it at room temperature for a couple of hours. Turn on the oven at 180 ° C, transfer the dough into a 23 cm long plum cake mold, with butter and flour. Brush the surface with milk and decorate with the granulated sugar. Cook in the hot oven for about 40 minutes.

Chicken strips

Ingredients

- 100 gr of chicken breast
- 50 gr of flour
- 10 gr of butter
- salt
- pepper

Preparation

1. To make the chicken strips in white wine, you must first of all cut the chicken breasts into irregular strips. Then put them inside a bowl and flour them.
2. When the operation is finished, put the butter in a large pan, then let it melt at a very low flame. Once the butter is melted, add the floured strips.
3. At this point let cook for a couple of minutes on a very lively flame. Add salt and pepper, then add the white wine. Cook the meat for two minutes. Then, put the lid on the pot that contains your chicken strips so as to evaporate the liquid and, when the sauce that accompanies it will be formed, turn off the heat. Conclude the preparation by letting the dish rest for a few minutes before serving.

Cheese and jam

Ingredients

- 4 types of cheese of your choice
- jam of your choice

Preparation

1. Cut 4 types of cheese and place them on the sides of a serving dish with only the grains in the center. If you have the possibility, put a small cup in the center with some autumn jam compost as well. This recipe is ideal for a fine dinner or as an appetizer with friends.

Day 7

French toast

Ingredients

- 2 slices of bread
- 2 eggs
- 10 gr of milk
- 10 gr of butter

Preparation

1. The French toast is a slightly richer solution, I usually use the classic slices of breaded, and when cooked I divide them in half, but it is fine to use simple bread cut into slices, better if stale.
2. Beat the eggs and milk, dip the slices of bread and put in the pan already hot and greased with butter. Cook a couple of minutes per side.
3. To freeze them I use the same procedure as the pancakes, and I prefer to offer them to the small ones simply sprinkled with a little sugar and cinnamon, which also has a strong antibacterial action, preventive for the cold season's ailments.

Tricolor salad

Ingredients

- Fresh cheese
- 2 tomatoes
- 2 zucchini
- oil
- salt pepper

- 2 marjoram leaves

Preparation

1. To prepare the tricolor salad with fresh cheese, cut the tomatoes into wedges and the zucchini into thin strips with a vegetable slicer. In a large bowl mix the zucchini and season with oil, salt, pepper and fresh marjoram leaves. Let the zucchini rest for about ten minutes in the cool. Then add the tomatoes and mix well. Serve the cheese accompanied by the vegetables prepared in this way.

Gorgonzola omelet

Ingredients

- 2 eggs
- 100 gr of gorgonzola
- cream cheese
- 10 gr of butter
- 100 gr of flour

Preparation

1. Prepare your gorgonzola omelet by separating egg whites and egg yolks. Add gorgonzola cheese to the yolks and season with white pepper. Add a pinch of salt to the egg whites and whisk them to the snow. Gently incorporate them into the cream cheese by mixing from bottom to top. Turn on the oven grill. Melt the butter in the pan. Pour in the egg mixture and cook for a couple of minutes on medium heat. When the omelet is golden in the lower part, slide it on a plate and place it under the grill to finish cooking. Serve the omelet gorgonzola well cooked, just out of the oven.

Chapter 2: Week 2

Day 1

Puff pastry treat

Ingredients

- 1 loaf of puff pastry
- sugar
- a pinch of cinnamon

Preparation

1. Roll out a loaf of puff pastry in a rectangular dough, sprinkle with sugar to which you have added a pinch of cinnamon and roll out with a rolling pin to make the sugar adhere well to the surfaces.
2. Roll the dough starting from the two sides until you get to the center. The result should be to have two cylinders wrapped around each other, joined to the center. Cut a lot of slices with a smooth blade knife.
3. Put the pieces on a baking sheet covered with parchment paper and bake in a preheated oven at 180 degrees.
4. Cook for about 15 minutes or until golden brown. Raise the puff pastry fans from the pan, turn them upside down, let them cool and serve.

Curry pasta

Ingredients

- 150 gr of pasta
- salt
- olive oil
- 1 tomato
- 100 gr of drained tuna
- 20 gr of curry

Preparation

1. To prepare curry pasta, you must first of all boil the water for the pasta.
2. Then add salt, melt the salt and pour the pasta.
3. Meanwhile, in a skillet, put a little extra virgin olive oil, then brown the garlic previously washed and crushed. When the garlic has turned blond, add the washed tomato, deprived of the seeds of the internal water and reduced into cubes.
4. Now everything is mixed, and the drained tuna is also added. Finally, cook for about 2 minutes. After the indicated time, melt the curry in half a glass of pasta cooking water.
5. Cook and mix the mixture until a creamy mixture is obtained.
6. Drain the pasta and pour it into the condiment pan.

Pasta with zucchini

Ingredients

- 150 gr of pasta
- 2 zucchini
- 10 gr of butter
- salt
- 100 gr of gorgonzola

Preparation

1. To make pasta with zucchini, you must first boil plenty of salted water. Wash, dry and cut the courgettes into slices, and chop the onion. Heat the butter in a large pan, pour the onion and let it dry, then add the zucchini and cook for a few minutes; season with salt and pepper.

2. When the water is boiling, pour the spaghetti, and as soon as it is bent, drain it with the help of kitchen tongs, taking care to keep the cooking water. Pour the spaghetti into the pan with the zucchini and cover with 3 ladles of cooking water; cut the gorgonzola cheese into cubes and put them aside. When the pasta is cooked, and the water is completely absorbed, add the cubes of Gorgonzola, carefully mixed until a velvety, creamy sauce that wraps the spaghetti is formed; if necessary, mix with very little cooking water. Serve your pasta with warm zucchini.

Day 2

Cocoa delight

Ingredients

- 1 egg
- 50 gr of whey
- sweetener
- 10 gr of hazelnuts
- 10 gr of crushed coconut
- bitter cocoa

Preparation

1. Mix the egg whites, the whey, and the sweetener. The mixture is poured into an anti-stick pan until a sort of omelet or crepe has formed (call it what you want).
2. Take the crepe and sprinkle over the minced hazelnuts and a part of the crushed coconut.
3. Close your fan-shaped crepe, sprinkle over the rest of the crushed coconut and sprinkle with the bitter cocoa.

Gnocchi with gorgonzola

Ingredients

- 100 gr of gnocchi
- 150 gr of gorgonzola
- salt
- olive oil

Preparation

1. To make gnocchi with gorgonzola, you will first have to take care of the seasoning. Take a non-stick frying pan with high

sides and let us melt the butter. Once the butter is melted, pour the Gorgonzola into a pan.

2. At this point let cook the two ingredients on low heat so that they blend together. Then, continuing to mix together the milk. Mix everything. Then season the sauce with salt and pepper. Let the mixture thicken by turning continuously.

3. At the end of the operation, dedicate yourself to cooking the gnocchi. Bring the water to a boil, add salt and add a drop of extra virgin olive oil.

4. Then cook the gnocchi inside. When the gnocchi rises to the surface, drain and season with the sauce previously prepared and stretched with a spoon of cooking water.

5. Once drained, stir in the gnocchi in a ready-made sauce. Serve your gnocchi hot.

Cream cheese

Ingredients

- 150 gr of gorgonzola
- 150 gr of mascarpone cheese
- 10 walnuts

Preparation

1. To make the cream cheese, mix well the Gorgonzola at room temperature with Mascarpone cheese.

2. Chop half the kernels of walnuts, add them to the mixture and stir. Then put the mixture in a small bowl, decorated with the remaining part of the walnuts and place in the fridge to rest. Your cream cheese will be perfect to spread on toasted bread or to be served with thinly sliced crudités, carrots, celery stalks or courgettes to taste.

Day 3

Sweet Treat

Ingredients

- 100 gr of raisins
- 10 gr of butter
- 1 egg
- 1 tablespoon of honey

Preparation

1. Soften the raisins in the Cointreau for about 20 minutes.
2. Cream the softened butter, then add the beaten egg and honey. Stir until it is creamy, then add the flour and baking powder and work until a soft dough is obtained. Squeeze the raisins and add to the mixture. With the dough obtained, make balls of dough that you will place on a baking sheet covered with paper ovens taking care to space the balls from each other. Cook the biscuits without sugar at 170 degrees for 15 minutes. Let them cool before lifting from the pan and serve.

Sardines

Ingredients

- 100 gr of sardines
- 1 lemon peel
- 1 lemon
- salt
- chopped parsley

Preparation

How is it best to consume sardines to fully exploit their nutritional properties? Baked with a sprinkling of lemon peel can be a useful and healthy alternative to the most famous fried version, especially for more frequent consumption.

1. Spice the sardines by removing the head towards the belly, to eliminate the entrails and the central spine, then pass them under running water and let them drain in a colander. Blot them well with absorbent paper and lay them on an oven lacquer in which you have previously added 1 tablespoon of oil.
2. Grate the rind of 1 untreated lemon directly on the sardines, add a pinch of salt and chopped parsley. Sprinkle with the remaining oil and bake at 200 ° C for 20 minutes or until complete cooking. Serve hot.

Toast and beans

Ingredients

- Bread
- shelled beans 100 gr
- 50 gr of cheese
- olive oil
- salt
- pepper

Preparation

1. Cut the bread into small squares and toast it under the grill. Meanwhile, shelled the beans (even their inner peel). Cut the cheese into cubes and put them in a large oven dish. Sprinkle all of extra virgin olive oil, salt, and pepper to your liking and last, before sitting on the table of the small croutons of bread.

Day 4

Pineapple treat

Ingredients

- 1 pineapple
- 1 lemon
- ginger
- 100 gr of ricotta

Preparation

1. Cut the slices of pineapple into small pieces, put them in a bowl with lemon juice and ginger, stir and leave to flavor
2. In the meantime, prepare the ricotta cream while working with the icing sugar and grated lemon peel.
3. Whip the cream and add it to the ricotta cream, then add 2/3 of the pineapple syrup. Gently mix the mousse until a smooth and homogeneous cream is obtained. Put a base of pineapple pieces in each bowl. Then cover with the ricotta and pineapple mousse.
4. Garnish each bowl with a few pieces of pineapple held part, then put in the fridge to cool for 1 hour before serving.

Mushroom cream

Ingredients

- 100 gr of porcini mushroom
- 10 gr of butter
- 100 gr of flour
- a pinch of salt
- minced parsley

Preparation

To make the cream of mushroom, you must first wash and clean the porcini mushrooms.

Slice and fry them with the butter. Then sprinkle the mixture with the flour and pour 1 liter of water.

At this point, leave the preparation on the fire until a thick cream has formed (it will take about 15 minutes).

Once obtained a cream of the right consistency, add the cream, a pinch of salt and the minced parsley. Continue to cook the dish for a few minutes. Then add a little bit of Gorgonzola (the amount depends on your taste and how much you want a more firm or more delicate dish).

Finally, serve the mushroom soup on toasted croutons. If you want, you can spread a veil of gorgonzola before serving.

Cheese pattern

Ingredients

- 4 different types of cheese
- 1 dish spoonful of jam or mustard

Preparation

1. Cut the cheeses into strips and arrange them in a radial pattern on a flat plate. In the middle of the dish 1 spoonful of each jam and mustard. Add the mustard with the Gorgonzola and the jams with the other cheeses

Day 5

Muffin with vegetables and cheese

Ingredients

- Different vegetables
- 2 eggs
- 100 gr of cheese

Preparation

A super easy low carb breakfast is vegetables, eggs, cheese, and muffins.
Here is how you can prepare them.

1. Spray a muffin pan with some oil. Scramble eggs with milk, cheese, and vegetables Pour a little mixture into the muffin mold. Bake at 200 degrees for 20 minutes.

Fennel salad

Ingredients

- 100 gr of fennel buds
- 1 mozzarella
- garlic
- olive oil
- salt
- vinegar
- pepper

Preparation

1. To prepare the fennel salad you must first wash, cleanse and reduce the fennel buds to julienne, then you have to take the mozzarella cheese and cut it into cubes.

2. Then dedicate yourself to the croutons. Take the croutons and rub them with the previously cleaned garlic cloves. Rub the slices into croutons until completely consumed.
3. Once the operation is complete, place the croutons on the bottom of a large salad bowl. At this point, pour over it, little by little and slowly, the extra virgin olive oil and the vinegar. Once the extra virgin olive oil and the vinegar have been poured, let the whole absorb.
4. So join us the julienne of fennel. Finally season with salt and pepper. Finish your salad by sprinkling it with the cheese cubes. Let it flavor and serve.

Healthy salad

Ingredients

- 100 gr of salad
- 100 gr of cheese
- 100 gr of bread

Preparation

1. Clean and wash the salad; take a type of cheese that you like, cut into cubes, and cut another one into strips, putting them on the bottom of the salad bowl. Cut the bread into slices and rub it with the garlic clove. Add everything in the salad bowl, season and serve.

Day 6

Donuts

Ingredients

- 2 eggs
- 50 gr of sugar
- 20 gr of oil
- 1 package of baking powder
- 100 gr of flour
- vanilla essence

Preparation

1. Whip the eggs with the sugar until you get a frothy mixture. Add the oil and then the water and the essence of vanilla.
2. Mix the flour with baking powder and lemon peel.
3. Add everything in the dough and continue to mount until you get a homogeneous mixture.
4. Pour the mixture into an oiled donuts mold.
5. Bake the donuts at 180 ° C in a preheated oven and cook for 40 minutes or until the toothpick is not ready with the toothpick test.
6. Allow the donuts to cool in the water, then turn it over a serving dish and sprinkle with icing sugar.

Lasagna with pesto

Ingredients

- 100 gr of pesto
- salt
- pepper
- lasagna dough

- bechamel sauce
- 50 gr of parmesan

Preparation

1. To make lasagna with pesto, you must, first of all, bring a bowl and mix inside it the béchamel with pesto, salt, and black pepper. Mix everything with a whisk, to prevent the formation of lumps.
2. At this point, pour a small amount of the mixture just prepared on the bottom of a medium pan or a baking dish and arrange the lasagna in order.
3. cover the pasta with the pesto and the béchamel sauce
4. Pour over the lasagna the béchamel sauce, a layer of cheese at will and, if you wish, put some grated Parmesan. Proceed in the same way until the last layer. Bake at 160 ° and cook in the oven until the lasagna with pesto turns slightly golden. When cooked, serve the hot nice dish.

Grilled aubergines

Ingredients

- 150 gr of aubergines
- 1 mozzarella
- 2 tomatoes

Preparation

1. Grill the aubergines and season with salt and pepper. Cut the mozzarella cheese into sticks and with the aubergines make the rolls with the mozzarella inside. Cut the tomatoes into wedges, season them and serve the rolls with the tomatoes on a serving plate.

Day 7

Apple treats

Ingredients

- puff pastry
- 5 apples
- 100 gr of sugar
- 50 gr of milk
- 20 gr of almond grains

Preparation

1. Cut the puff pastry into 6 rectangles. Peel the apples and cut thin slices.
2. Arrange 6 slices of apple in the center of each rectangle of pastry, overlapping one another slightly.
3. Melt the sugar in a small bowl with the milk and with it brush the edges of puff pastry free (if you prefer you can also use an egg to brush the puff pastry)
4. Melt the jam in a thick-bottomed saucepan and brush the surface of the apples with it.
5. Cover each apple puff pastry with almond grains.
6. Bake the pasty in an oven already hot and cook at 180 degrees for about 10 minutes.
7. Allow the apple puffs to cool and serve.

Ricotta and spinach ravioli

Ingredients

- 2 eggs
- 100 gr of ricotta
- 100 gr of spinach
- salt
- pepper
- 200 gr of flour

Preparation

1. To make ricotta and spinach ravioli, you must first sift the flour on the pastry board, place it in a fountain and pour the beaten eggs inside, a pinch of salt and a spoonful of warm water. Mix everything with the aid of a fork, then continue to knead the ingredients for at least 10 minutes. The dough should be smooth and elastic.
2. Once ready, pick up the dough giving it the shape of a ball and wrap it in a sheet of transparent film for food. Leave it to rest for about 60 minutes.
3. In the meantime, take care of the filling: clean and wash the spinach. Then cook for a few minutes with only the water left over from the wash, then drain them, squeeze them well in your hands, then chop finely with the crescent.
4. At this point, pour them in a bowl and add the ricotta cheese, the eggs, the nutmeg, the salt and the pepper. Mix everything carefully until you have a smooth and homogeneous mixture.
5. At the end of the operation, divide the pasta previously prepared into four pieces and, using the machine to pull the dough, make a thin strip from each one. Then place on the long side of the strip small piles of ricotta and spinach the size of a cherry (you can help with a teaspoon). Place them at a distance of 4 centimeters from each other. Once the strip of

dough has been used to lay the filling, proceed to fold the flap of free pasta, so as to cover the filling balls well. At this point press with your fingers around the filling so as to let the air out and to seal well your ricotta and spinach ravioli. Then cut the ravioli with the toothed wheel and, as they are ready, place them on a floured plate.

Avocado passion

Ingredients

- 1 avocado
- 1 pineapple
- 100 gr of ricotta
- 1 tablespoon of salt

Preparation

1. Clean the avocado, open it and cut into slices, flip endive and thinly slice the pineapple and mango. Arrange the endive leaves on the bottom of the serving dish, in a radial pattern, then overlay the avocado, the pineapple. Cover with a sauce prepared by softening the ricotta cheese with pineapple juice or water and salt. Place the pre-cooked and shelled prawns in the center and serve cold.

Conclusion

Congratulations! And thank for making it through to the end of this book, let's hope it was informative and able to provide you with all of the tools you need to achieve your goals whatever they may be.

** Remember to use your link to claim your 3 FREE Cookbooks on Health, Fitness & Dieting Instantly

https://bit.ly/2MkqTit

Printed in Great Britain
by Amazon

24322655R00030